# This Pregnancy Journal Belongs to

_____

_____

I am _____ years old.

This is my _____ pregnancy

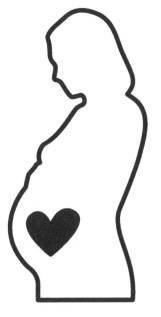

# First-time experiences

## When?

Positive pregnancy test
_____
_____
_____

Ultrasound
_____
_____
_____

Food craving
_____
_____
_____

Felt baby kick
_____
_____
_____

Hiccups
_____
_____
_____

Felt contraction
_____
_____
_____

Heard heartbeat
_____
_____
_____

Other memorable first time
_____
_____
_____

## Names for our baby

Girl

Boy

Why we love them?

# First Ultrasound

First photo

| Date | Weight | Length | Note |
|------|--------|--------|------|
|      |        |        |      |

Our Reaction

Our Family Reaction

# Appointments

| Date | Time | Place | Reason |
|------|------|-------|--------|
|  |  |  |  |
|  |  |  |  |
|  |  |  |  |
|  |  |  |  |
|  |  |  |  |
|  |  |  |  |
|  |  |  |  |
|  |  |  |  |
|  |  |  |  |
|  |  |  |  |
|  |  |  |  |
|  |  |  |  |
|  |  |  |  |
|  |  |  |  |

# Appointments

| Date | Time | Place | Reason |
|------|------|-------|--------|
|      |      |       |        |
|      |      |       |        |
|      |      |       |        |
|      |      |       |        |
|      |      |       |        |
|      |      |       |        |
|      |      |       |        |
|      |      |       |        |
|      |      |       |        |
|      |      |       |        |
|      |      |       |        |
|      |      |       |        |
|      |      |       |        |

# Appointments

| Date | Time | Place | Reason |
|------|------|-------|--------|
|      |      |       |        |
|      |      |       |        |
|      |      |       |        |
|      |      |       |        |
|      |      |       |        |
|      |      |       |        |
|      |      |       |        |
|      |      |       |        |
|      |      |       |        |
|      |      |       |        |
|      |      |       |        |
|      |      |       |        |

# Appointments

| Date | Time | Place | Reason |
|------|------|-------|--------|
|      |      |       |        |
|      |      |       |        |
|      |      |       |        |
|      |      |       |        |
|      |      |       |        |
|      |      |       |        |
|      |      |       |        |
|      |      |       |        |
|      |      |       |        |
|      |      |       |        |
|      |      |       |        |
|      |      |       |        |
|      |      |       |        |
|      |      |       |        |

Mood

Sleep

☆ ☆ ☆ ☆ ☆

Symptoms

I feel the best when:

Moment to remember

I feel the worst when:

How I feel?

Food that calms my belly

Belly measurements/Weight

Food that upset my belly

| Vitamins | M | T | W | T | F | S | S |
|----------|---|---|---|---|---|---|---|
|          |   |   |   |   |   |   |   |
|          |   |   |   |   |   |   |   |
|          |   |   |   |   |   |   |   |
|          |   |   |   |   |   |   |   |

## WEEK 2

Mood

_____

Sleep

☆ ☆ ☆ ☆ ☆

Symptoms

I feel the best when:

Moment to remember

I feel the worst when:

How I feel?

Food that calms my belly

Belly measurements/Weight

Food that upset my belly

| Vitamins | M | T | W | T | F | S | S |
|----------|---|---|---|---|---|---|---|
|          |   |   |   |   |   |   |   |
|          |   |   |   |   |   |   |   |
|          |   |   |   |   |   |   |   |
|          |   |   |   |   |   |   |   |

Mood

Sleep

☆ ☆ ☆ ☆ ☆

Symptoms

I feel the best when:

Moment to remember

I feel the worst when:

How I feel?

Food that calms my belly

Belly measurements/Weight

Food that upset my belly

| Vitamins | M | T | W | T | F | S | S |
|---|---|---|---|---|---|---|---|
| | | | | | | | |
| | | | | | | | |
| | | | | | | | |
| | | | | | | | |

Mood

Sleep
☆ ☆ ☆ ☆ ☆

Symptoms

I feel the best when:

Moment to remember

I feel the worst when:

How I feel?

Food that calms my belly

Belly measurements/Weight

Food that upset my belly

| Vitamins | M | T | W | T | F | S | S |
|---|---|---|---|---|---|---|---|
|  |  |  |  |  |  |  |  |
|  |  |  |  |  |  |  |  |
|  |  |  |  |  |  |  |  |
|  |  |  |  |  |  |  |  |

Mood

Sleep

☆ ☆ ☆ ☆ ☆

Symptoms

I feel the best when:

Moment to remember

I feel the worst when:

How I feel?

Food that calms my belly

Belly measurements/Weight

Food that upset my belly

| Vitamins | M | T | W | T | F | S | S |
|---|---|---|---|---|---|---|---|
| | | | | | | | |
| | | | | | | | |
| | | | | | | | |
| | | | | | | | |

## Mood

## Sleep

☆ ☆ ☆ ☆ ☆

## Symptoms

## I feel the best when:

## Moment to remember

## I feel the worst when:

## How I feel?

## Food that calms my belly

## Belly measurements/Weight

## Food that upset my belly

| Vitamins | M | T | W | T | F | S | S |
|---|---|---|---|---|---|---|---|
|  |  |  |  |  |  |  |  |
|  |  |  |  |  |  |  |  |
|  |  |  |  |  |  |  |  |
|  |  |  |  |  |  |  |  |
|  |  |  |  |  |  |  |  |

Mood

Sleep
☆ ☆ ☆ ☆ ☆

Symptoms

I feel the best when:

Moment to remember

I feel the worst when:

How I feel?

Food that calms my belly

Belly measurements/Weight

Food that upset my belly

| Vitamins | M | T | W | T | F | S | S |
|----------|---|---|---|---|---|---|---|
|          |   |   |   |   |   |   |   |
|          |   |   |   |   |   |   |   |
|          |   |   |   |   |   |   |   |
|          |   |   |   |   |   |   |   |

Mood

Sleep

☆ ☆ ☆ ☆ ☆

Symptoms

I feel the best when:

Moment to remember

I feel the worst when:

How I feel?

Food that calms my belly

Belly measurements/Weight

Food that upset my belly

| Vitamins | M | T | W | T | F | S | S |
|---|---|---|---|---|---|---|---|
| | | | | | | | |
| | | | | | | | |
| | | | | | | | |
| | | | | | | | |

Mood

Sleep
☆ ☆ ☆ ☆ ☆

Symptoms

I feel the best when:

Moment to remember

I feel the worst when:

How I feel?

Food that calms my belly

Belly measurements/Weight

Food that upset my belly

| Vitamins | M | T | W | T | F | S | S |
|----------|---|---|---|---|---|---|---|
|          |   |   |   |   |   |   |   |
|          |   |   |   |   |   |   |   |
|          |   |   |   |   |   |   |   |
|          |   |   |   |   |   |   |   |

Mood

Sleep

☆ ☆ ☆ ☆ ☆

Symptoms

I feel the best when:

Moment to remember

I feel the worst when:

How I feel?

Food that calms my belly

Belly measurements/Weight

Food that upset my belly

| Vitamins | M | T | W | T | F | S | S |
|----------|---|---|---|---|---|---|---|
|          |   |   |   |   |   |   |   |
|          |   |   |   |   |   |   |   |
|          |   |   |   |   |   |   |   |
|          |   |   |   |   |   |   |   |

Mood

Sleep
☆ ☆ ☆ ☆ ☆

Symptoms

I feel the best when:

Moment to remember

I feel the worst when:

How I feel?

Food that calms my belly

Belly measurements/Weight

Food that upset my belly

| Vitamins | M | T | W | T | F | S | S |
|---|---|---|---|---|---|---|---|
| | | | | | | | |
| | | | | | | | |
| | | | | | | | |
| | | | | | | | |
| | | | | | | | |

Mood

Sleep

☆ ☆ ☆ ☆ ☆

Symptoms

I feel the best when:

Moment to remember

I feel the worst when:

How I feel?

Food that calms my belly

Belly measurements/Weight

Food that upset my belly

| Vitamins | M | T | W | T | F | S | S |
|---|---|---|---|---|---|---|---|
|  |  |  |  |  |  |  |  |
|  |  |  |  |  |  |  |  |
|  |  |  |  |  |  |  |  |
|  |  |  |  |  |  |  |  |

Mood

Sleep
☆ ☆ ☆ ☆ ☆

Symptoms

I feel the best when:

Moment to remember

I feel the worst when:

How I feel?

Food that calms my belly

Belly measurements/Weight

Food that upset my belly

| Vitamins | M | T | W | T | F | S | S |
|---|---|---|---|---|---|---|---|
| | | | | | | | |
| | | | | | | | |
| | | | | | | | |
| | | | | | | | |

## Mood

## Sleep

☆ ☆ ☆ ☆ ☆

## Symptoms

## I feel the best when:

## Moment to remember

## I feel the worst when:

## How I feel?

## Food that calms my belly

## Belly measurements/Weight

## Food that upset my belly

| Vitamins | M | T | W | T | F | S | S |
|----------|---|---|---|---|---|---|---|
|          |   |   |   |   |   |   |   |
|          |   |   |   |   |   |   |   |
|          |   |   |   |   |   |   |   |
|          |   |   |   |   |   |   |   |

Mood

Sleep
☆ ☆ ☆ ☆ ☆

Symptoms

I feel the best when:

Moment to remember

I feel the worst when:

How I feel?

Food that calms my belly

Belly measurements/Weight

Food that upset my belly

| Vitamins | M | T | W | T | F | S | S |
|----------|---|---|---|---|---|---|---|
|          |   |   |   |   |   |   |   |
|          |   |   |   |   |   |   |   |
|          |   |   |   |   |   |   |   |
|          |   |   |   |   |   |   |   |

Mood

Sleep

☆ ☆ ☆ ☆ ☆

_____

Symptoms

I feel the best when:

Moment to remember

I feel the worst when:

How I feel?

Food that calms my belly

Belly measurements/Weight

Food that upset my belly

| Vitamins | M | T | W | T | F | S | S |
|---|---|---|---|---|---|---|---|
|  |  |  |  |  |  |  |  |
|  |  |  |  |  |  |  |  |
|  |  |  |  |  |  |  |  |
|  |  |  |  |  |  |  |  |

## WEEK 17

### Mood

### Sleep
☆ ☆ ☆ ☆ ☆

### Symptoms

### I feel the best when:

### Moment to remember

### I feel the worst when:

### How I feel?

### Food that calms my belly

### Belly measurements/Weight

### Food that upset my belly

| Vitamins | M | T | W | T | F | S | S |
|---|---|---|---|---|---|---|---|
|  |  |  |  |  |  |  |  |
|  |  |  |  |  |  |  |  |
|  |  |  |  |  |  |  |  |
|  |  |  |  |  |  |  |  |

Mood

Sleep
☆ ☆ ☆ ☆ ☆

Symptoms

I feel the best when:

Moment to remember

I feel the worst when:

How I feel?

Food that calms my belly

Belly measurements/Weight

Food that upset my belly

| Vitamins | M | T | W | T | F | S | S |
|----------|---|---|---|---|---|---|---|
|          |   |   |   |   |   |   |   |
|          |   |   |   |   |   |   |   |
|          |   |   |   |   |   |   |   |
|          |   |   |   |   |   |   |   |
|          |   |   |   |   |   |   |   |

Mood

Sleep

☆ ☆ ☆ ☆ ☆

Symptoms

I feel the best when:

Moment to remember

I feel the worst when:

How I feel?

Food that calms my belly

Belly measurements/Weight

Food that upset my belly

| Vitamins | M | T | W | T | F | S | S |
|----------|---|---|---|---|---|---|---|
|          |   |   |   |   |   |   |   |
|          |   |   |   |   |   |   |   |
|          |   |   |   |   |   |   |   |
|          |   |   |   |   |   |   |   |

## Mood

## Sleep

☆ ☆ ☆ ☆ ☆

## Symptoms

## I feel the best when:

## Moment to remember

## I feel the worst when:

## How I feel?

## Food that calms my belly

## Belly measurements/Weight

## Food that upset my belly

| Vitamins | M | T | W | T | F | S | S |
|---|---|---|---|---|---|---|---|
| | | | | | | | |
| | | | | | | | |
| | | | | | | | |
| | | | | | | | |

Mood

Sleep
☆ ☆ ☆ ☆ ☆

Symptoms

I feel the best when:

Moment to remember

I feel the worst when:

How I feel?

Food that calms my belly

Belly measurements/Weight

Food that upset my belly

| Vitamins | M | T | W | T | F | S | S |
|----------|---|---|---|---|---|---|---|
|          |   |   |   |   |   |   |   |
|          |   |   |   |   |   |   |   |
|          |   |   |   |   |   |   |   |
|          |   |   |   |   |   |   |   |

## Mood

## Sleep
☆ ☆ ☆ ☆ ☆

## Symptoms

### I feel the best when:

## Moment to remember

### I feel the worst when:

## How I feel?

### Food that calms my belly

## Belly measurements/Weight

### Food that upset my belly

| Vitamins | M | T | W | T | F | S | S |
|---|---|---|---|---|---|---|---|
| | | | | | | | |
| | | | | | | | |
| | | | | | | | |
| | | | | | | | |
| | | | | | | | |

## WEEK 23

**Mood**

**Sleep**
☆ ☆ ☆ ☆ ☆

**Symptoms**

**I feel the best when:**

**Moment to remember**

**I feel the worst when:**

**How I feel?**

**Food that calms my belly**

**Belly measurements/Weight**

**Food that upset my belly**

| Vitamins | M | T | W | T | F | S | S |
|---|---|---|---|---|---|---|---|
|  |  |  |  |  |  |  |  |
|  |  |  |  |  |  |  |  |
|  |  |  |  |  |  |  |  |
|  |  |  |  |  |  |  |  |

## Mood

## Sleep

☆ ☆ ☆ ☆ ☆

## Symptoms

## I feel the best when:

## Moment to remember

## I feel the worst when:

## How I feel?

## Food that calms my belly

## Belly measurements/Weight

## Food that upset my belly

| Vitamins | M | T | W | T | F | S | S |
|---|---|---|---|---|---|---|---|
|  |  |  |  |  |  |  |  |
|  |  |  |  |  |  |  |  |
|  |  |  |  |  |  |  |  |
|  |  |  |  |  |  |  |  |

Mood

Sleep
☆☆☆☆☆

Symptoms

I feel the best when:

Moment to remember

I feel the worst when:

How I feel?

Food that calms my belly

Belly measurements/Weight

Food that upset my belly

| Vitamins | M | T | W | T | F | S | S |
|---|---|---|---|---|---|---|---|
| | | | | | | | |
| | | | | | | | |
| | | | | | | | |
| | | | | | | | |

Mood

Sleep
☆☆☆☆☆

Symptoms

I feel the best when:

Moment to remember

I feel the worst when:

How I feel?

Food that calms my belly

Belly measurements/Weight

Food that upset my belly

| Vitamins | M | T | W | T | F | S | S |
|----------|---|---|---|---|---|---|---|
|          |   |   |   |   |   |   |   |
|          |   |   |   |   |   |   |   |
|          |   |   |   |   |   |   |   |
|          |   |   |   |   |   |   |   |

Mood

Sleep

☆ ☆ ☆ ☆ ☆

Symptoms

I feel the best when:

Moment to remember

I feel the worst when:

How I feel?

Food that calms my belly

Belly measurements/Weight

Food that upset my belly

| Vitamins | M | T | W | T | F | S | S |
|---|---|---|---|---|---|---|---|
|  |  |  |  |  |  |  |  |
|  |  |  |  |  |  |  |  |
|  |  |  |  |  |  |  |  |
|  |  |  |  |  |  |  |  |

## Mood

_____

## Sleep

☆☆☆☆☆

## Symptoms

## I feel the best when:

## Moment to remember

## I feel the worst when:

## How I feel?

## Food that calms my belly

## Belly measurements/Weight

## Food that upset my belly

| Vitamins | M | T | W | T | F | S | S |
|---|---|---|---|---|---|---|---|
|  |  |  |  |  |  |  |  |
|  |  |  |  |  |  |  |  |
|  |  |  |  |  |  |  |  |
|  |  |  |  |  |  |  |  |

Mood

Sleep
☆ ☆ ☆ ☆ ☆

Symptoms

I feel the best when:

Moment to remember

I feel the worst when:

How I feel?

Food that calms my belly

Belly measurements/Weight

Food that upset my belly

| Vitamins | M | T | W | T | F | S | S |
|----------|---|---|---|---|---|---|---|
|          |   |   |   |   |   |   |   |
|          |   |   |   |   |   |   |   |
|          |   |   |   |   |   |   |   |
|          |   |   |   |   |   |   |   |

Mood

Sleep

☆ ☆ ☆ ☆ ☆

Symptoms

I feel the best when:

Moment to remember

I feel the worst when:

How I feel?

Food that calms my belly

Belly measurements/Weight

Food that upset my belly

| Vitamins | M | T | W | T | F | S | S |
|---|---|---|---|---|---|---|---|
|  |  |  |  |  |  |  |  |
|  |  |  |  |  |  |  |  |
|  |  |  |  |  |  |  |  |
|  |  |  |  |  |  |  |  |

Mood

Sleep
☆ ☆ ☆ ☆ ☆

Symptoms

I feel the best when:

Moment to remember

I feel the worst when:

How I feel?

Food that calms my belly

Belly measurements/Weight

Food that upset my belly

| Vitamins | M | T | W | T | F | S | S |
|---|---|---|---|---|---|---|---|
| | | | | | | | |
| | | | | | | | |
| | | | | | | | |
| | | | | | | | |

Mood

Sleep

☆☆☆☆☆

Symptoms

I feel the best when:

Moment to remember

I feel the worst when:

How I feel?

Food that calms my belly

Belly measurements/Weight

Food that upset my belly

| Vitamins | M | T | W | T | F | S | S |
|---|---|---|---|---|---|---|---|
|  |  |  |  |  |  |  |  |
|  |  |  |  |  |  |  |  |
|  |  |  |  |  |  |  |  |
|  |  |  |  |  |  |  |  |

## Mood

_____

_____

## Sleep

☆ ☆ ☆ ☆ ☆

## Symptoms

## I feel the best when:

## Moment to remember

## I feel the worst when:

## How I feel?

## Food that calms my belly

## Belly measurements/Weight

## Food that upset my belly

| Vitamins | M | T | W | T | F | S | S |
|----------|---|---|---|---|---|---|---|
|          |   |   |   |   |   |   |   |
|          |   |   |   |   |   |   |   |
|          |   |   |   |   |   |   |   |
|          |   |   |   |   |   |   |   |

## Mood

_____

## Sleep

☆ ☆ ☆ ☆ ☆

### Symptoms

### I feel the best when:

### Moment to remember

### I feel the worst when:

### How I feel?

### Food that calms my belly

### Belly measurements/Weight

### Food that upset my belly

| Vitamins | M | T | W | T | F | S | S |
|---|---|---|---|---|---|---|---|
|  |  |  |  |  |  |  |  |
|  |  |  |  |  |  |  |  |
|  |  |  |  |  |  |  |  |
|  |  |  |  |  |  |  |  |
|  |  |  |  |  |  |  |  |

Mood

Sleep
☆ ☆ ☆ ☆ ☆

Symptoms

I feel the best when:

Moment to remember

I feel the worst when:

How I feel?

Food that calms my belly

Belly measurements/Weight

Food that upset my belly

| Vitamins | M | T | W | T | F | S | S |
|---|---|---|---|---|---|---|---|
| | | | | | | | |
| | | | | | | | |
| | | | | | | | |
| | | | | | | | |

Mood

Sleep
☆ ☆ ☆ ☆ ☆

Symptoms

I feel the best when:

Moment to remember

I feel the worst when:

How I feel?

Food that calms my belly

Belly measurements/Weight

Food that upset my belly

| Vitamins | M | T | W | T | F | S | S |
|---|---|---|---|---|---|---|---|
|  |  |  |  |  |  |  |  |
|  |  |  |  |  |  |  |  |
|  |  |  |  |  |  |  |  |
|  |  |  |  |  |  |  |  |

Mood

Sleep
☆ ☆ ☆ ☆ ☆

Symptoms

I feel the best when:

Moment to remember

I feel the worst when:

How I feel?

Food that calms my belly

Belly measurements/Weight

Food that upset my belly

| Vitamins | M | T | W | T | F | S | S |
|----------|---|---|---|---|---|---|---|
|          |   |   |   |   |   |   |   |
|          |   |   |   |   |   |   |   |
|          |   |   |   |   |   |   |   |
|          |   |   |   |   |   |   |   |

## Mood

_____

## Sleep

☆ ☆ ☆ ☆ ☆

## Symptoms

## I feel the best when:

## Moment to remember

## I feel the worst when:

## How I feel?

## Food that calms my belly

## Belly measurements/Weight

## Food that upset my belly

| Vitamins | M | T | W | T | F | S | S |
|---|---|---|---|---|---|---|---|
| | | | | | | | |
| | | | | | | | |
| | | | | | | | |
| | | | | | | | |

Mood

Sleep
☆☆☆☆☆

Symptoms

I feel the best when:

Moment to remember

I feel the worst when:

How I feel?

Food that calms my belly

Belly measurements/Weight

Food that upset my belly

| Vitamins | M | T | W | T | F | S | S |
|----------|---|---|---|---|---|---|---|
|          |   |   |   |   |   |   |   |
|          |   |   |   |   |   |   |   |
|          |   |   |   |   |   |   |   |
|          |   |   |   |   |   |   |   |

Mood

Sleep

☆☆☆☆☆

Symptoms

I feel the best when:

Moment to remember

I feel the worst when:

How I feel?

Food that calms my belly

Belly measurements/Weight

Food that upset my belly

| Vitamins | M | T | W | T | F | S | S |
|----------|---|---|---|---|---|---|---|
|          |   |   |   |   |   |   |   |
|          |   |   |   |   |   |   |   |
|          |   |   |   |   |   |   |   |
|          |   |   |   |   |   |   |   |

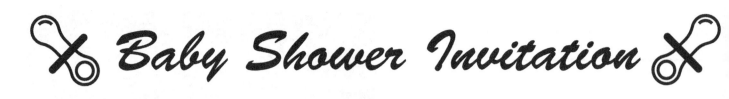

# Baby Shower Invitation

| Date/Time | Location | Thrown by |
|---|---|---|
| | | |

| Favorite Gifts | Favorite moments |
|---|---|
| | |

## Guests list

_____

_____

_____

_____

_____

_____

_____

_____

_____

# Baby Shower Invitation

# Almost time

## We are most excited for

## We are most nervous for

## What have I enjoyed most about being pregnant?

# My Labor

**Date labor began on**

**Place labor began on**

**Total hours in labor**

**Who came to visit?**

**Special healthcare workers to remember**

**Thoughts & Feelings**

# Notes

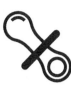 # Notes

# Notes

# Notes

# Notes

# Notes

# Notes

# Notes

# Notes

# Notes

# Notes

# Notes

# Notes

# Notes

# Notes

# Notes

# Notes

# Notes

# Notes

# Notes

# Notes

# Notes

# Notes

# Notes

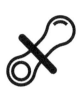

# Notes

# Notes

# Notes

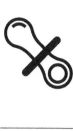

# Notes

# Notes

# Notes

# Notes

# Notes

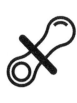

# Notes

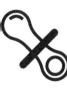

# Notes

# Notes

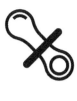# Notes

# Notes

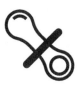

# Notes

# Notes

# Notes

# Notes

# Notes

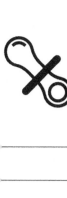

# Notes

# Notes

# Notes

# Notes

# Notes

# Notes

# Notes